One Hip Book

by

Mike Masterson

authorHOUSE™

1663 LIBERTY DRIVE, SUITE 200
BLOOMINGTON, INDIANA 47403
(800) 839-8640
WWW.AUTHORHOUSE.COM

First published by AuthorHouse 09/27/04

ISBN: 1-4184-7250-6 (e)
ISBN: 1-4184-7249-2 (sc)

Printed in the United States of America
Bloomington, Indiana

This book is printed on acid-free paper.

Dedication

*For my sweetheart compan-
ion and soulmate, Judith,
the best private duty nurse any man
could hope to have, and my beloved
son, Brandon and daughter, Anna. And
with appreciation and all due credit to
The Arkansas Democrat-Gazette. The
views expressed herein are solely those
of the author based on his personal experience and viewpoints. Any prospective hip replacement candidates should
always consult with their physicians

for professional medical advice. An updated list of MIS Zimmer-qualified surgeons can be found on the Internet at www.pacewithlife.com

ONE HIP BOOK

By Mike Masterson

*A nationally acclaimed journalist
explains
what it was like to anticipate, undergo
and successfully emerge from a
minimally-invasive
Zimmer - technique total hip
replacement surgery*

Feeling Your Pain

So you're considering having that aching bad hip replaced with an artificial one. Well, you've found the right book if you're looking for someone who faced, endured and emerged from the ordeal. In fact, you and I likely have much in common, whether it is osteoarthritis or some other disease that has left you considering a mini-incision replacement.

I understand all the thoughts and personal concerns you are having, perhaps better than your surgeon or anyone close to you. I've lived the many worrisome moments. And because I understand them so well, I decided I had to write this account with you in mind.

I am a journalist, a person whose purpose in his life and career is to explain to others what I feel, see and discover. Following my experiences with this surgery, I knew I would write about everything surrounding it, hoping to help others realize they are normal in their concerns, and to separate fact from fear and anxiety.

"One Hip Book," is based solely on my *adventure*, so to speak, with the Zimmer Corporation's MIS (Minimally Invasive Surgery) technique. The good news you'll discover, as you read deeper into these words, is that if I were to face the ordeal of a hip replacement again, I would do so without a shred of worry or fear. In fact, let's begin by talking about that fear.

The late Franklin D. Roosevelt reminded us in 1932 that we, "have nothing to fear but fear itself." Before his untimely death, singer John Denver also wrote how all our fears - even at their most intense - at their zeniths, mean nothing. Reassuring words, indeed. But when you're facing the replacement of a God-given hip with robotic devices forged of metal, ceramic or plastic - and when you know your leg is about to be amputated before being restored, I understand that fear and anxiety become a natural part of the process.

If this scenario fits your circumstances - if you're considering having a diseased hip replaced and feeling apprehensive over the uncertainty of it all, then this book is a must-read. Hopefully it will help bring peace to a troubled mind. Believe me, I know how dire it sounds just to hear a doctor utter the words "total hip replacement."

There is stark finality to such a sobering phrase that it makes many of us want to turn tail and grab for extra doses of our preferred anti-inflammatory prescription. That's how I felt when a general practitioner pronounced my sentence. It was the inevitable consequence of 56 years of overstuffing supersized meals that layered damaging tonnage on both hips.

I vividly recall the day. My good-natured general practitioner, Dr. Larry Tuttle, here in Fayetteville, Arkansas, held the X-Ray of my right hip tightly against the light box. He examined it only a few seconds before jabbing a forefinger toward my diseased joint. " Well, it's obvious you've got osteoarthritis right there in that joint. It's already pretty extensive, in fact. See all this bone rubbing against bone where your cartilage has worn away? And, Mike, I hate to tell you this, but that missing cartilage won't re-grow itself."

"That bad pain you've been feeling in the hip and deep inside your groin is being caused by the hip's femoral head continually rubbing against the cup that holds it," he continued, roughly outlining the affected area with a casual wave of his hand. Then came his most bone-chilling sentence. "You know, the only remedy for this incurable condition is (here's the first time I heard the phrase) a *total hip replacement*." All mincing of medical jargon aside, that meant literally cutting off my leg - a rather permanent condition by my simple layman's analysis.

And so it came to pass on that winter's day this Ozark's born arthritic officially launched his all-out counterattack to avoid hip arthroplasty. I preferred using this medically-vague *arthroplasty* term, since it conjured more an image of medical repair than of a wholesale replacement. If it meant I had to gulp down potent prescription pain medications and exercise constantly to shed pounds from my six-foot, 265-pound frame, then that's what I'd do. I simply could not get my mind around having my natural hip cut out and replaced with some cold, artificial version of God's handiwork.

Interestingly, in a later discussion, my orthopedic surgeon, would explain how the emotional impact of losing any body part can be compared with the predictable stages of loss described in the late Dr. Elizabeth Kubler Ross' renown book entitled "Death and Dying."

First I could expect the denial stage, followed by anger, then bargaining, despair and, finally, acceptance. In the months ahead, I did, in fact, pass through each phase. And you most likely will, too, as this little book explains. I would come over the ensuing weeks and months also to see replacing my hip as much in spiritual as I did physical terms.

After all, I reasoned, I was not really losing any of "me," by this replacement, any more than had I lost an arm or a tooth for that matter. The fundamental "me" that becomes conscious of itself for a brief period in this strange world is something much more mysterious and profound than any temporary body part that happens to carry my name.

My Denial

As good fortune would have it, I was one of those mid-50's Baby Boomers who'd been lucky enough to somehow avoid hospitals all those years. That seeming invincibility made me feel as though this disease that appeared from out of nowhere couldn't possibly be destroying my hip joint. Nope, not Mike's hip. I began a regimen of pills and a regular exercise routine complete with a personal trainer.

I stocked my medicine cabinet with bottles of triple-strength Glucosamine, Chondroitin and MSM. Then I began swallowing those horse pills twice each day. I was man enough, by God, to lick a crippling disease I'd always believed afflicted only the aged. At least that's what all the TV ads had taught me.

I also jumped face-first into muscle and tendon-stretching Pilates sessions twice a week to accompany workouts on the assorted weight machines. This had become all-out warfare - my personal D-Day invasion - and I was determined to win by overwhelming the enemy. I didn't even care to hear about the gritty details of hip replacement surgery. That, to me, was tantamount to treason and surrendering conquered territory.

This comfortable state of denial and my well-intentioned assault continued for months. But with each passing week, I also felt the grinding aches in my joint and groin relentlessly increasing. I soon learned how the groin pain emanating from the deep inner-thigh is often a tell-tale sign of osteoarthritis in the hip. My once-respectable golf game had steadily degenerated to the point where any balance was lost in wild, swaying lunges from above the waist.

I found I could not longer shift weight effectively through the ball, or use my legs properly. It just hurt too much. And, besides, I was trying my best to deny and ignore the constant pain. By the spring of 2003, my four-ball tournament partner,

Dave Fulton, who'd already had two hips replaced in the traditional manner, was jokingly referring to me as "the best golf partner he'd ever had on one leg." It got some big laughs around the club house.

Anger

I was smiling at his joke on the outside. But deep in my heart, I was steadily and inexorably coming face-to-face with reality. And it was making me mad as hell. This damn disease was winning despite my very best efforts. In desperation, I began researching the Internet for research into the possible regeneration of the cartilage and sonovial fluid that had somehow evaporated from my hip joint.

It just made sense that one day, hopefully soon, some brilliant medical researcher would discover a way to replace these worn-out natural joint cushions, especially with osteoarthritis becoming so prevalent in today's aging society.

In fact, I did discover one advertisement in a flight magazine that touted a series of supposedly regenerative injections available at some South Florida clinic near the beach. The rather convincing advertisement claimed these shots helped re-grow the lost cartilage in diseased hips. With elevated hopes, I phoned the clinic.

I came away from that 10-minute discussion feeling both uncertain and unconvinced. Although this clinic offered hope (perhaps misplaced), its injections cost hundreds of dollars for each non-guaranteed treatment. On top of that, patients had to provide transportation to and from South Florida while financing a week of lodging - investments based solely on desperate hopes.

I searched the Internet once again but couldn't locate any credible medical sources to verify the legitimacy of this treatment without guarantees. Finally, I abandoned the idea altogether as financially and practically unfeasible. Florida is a long way from Fayetteville and Northwest Arkansas. And I was wary that - with the retiree population that comprises much of South Florida region - this treatment could also have been more a tactic for reaping profit from false promises and promotions than curing the crippling effects of osteoarthritis.

With each passing week I slowly began entertaining the distasteful and unsettling prospect of traditional surgery. Surprisingly, I discovered many people I knew, like my friend Dave Fulton, already had undergone this long-form operation, followed by months of recovery and rehabilitation. In my community over the years, hundreds of men and women had experienced this method.

Each one I came to speak with said they ultimately were thankful they'd had their replacements, even as radical as the traditional 12 to 14-inch cut through their hip muscles had been. Some said they still didn't feel they were back to functioning near 100 percent even two years after their surgeries. All the while, my own discomfort was intensifying week by week. It reached the point where I would quickly seek out the first chair in any room. Just the act of lying in bed often triggered the grinding ache that by then had become as much a part of life as blinking and breathing.

Others I knew in the community were facing the same decision that I was, caused either by osteoarthritis or a condition known as Avascular Necrosis which methodically eats away the hip's femoral head until it no longer fits inside the cup. It became increasingly apparent that arthritis and other insidious diseases of the hip and knee joints are becoming more common than any of us Baby Boomers ever realized. We had stacked too many years and excess pounds on our aging joints for them to endure and function properly over time. Like a swelling balloon finally will pop, something inside finally just had to give. And believe me, these crucial joints are giving out by the millions as society ages.

The growing scourge of joint disease had been quietly spreading its misery right beneath our collective belly buttons over the past decade. I'd venture to say as you read these words that you - like me - are surrounded by others in your neighborhoods and communities who have undergone traditional joint replacement surgeries.

You just never were aware of it because their problems weren't impacting on you. I've always said the best way to understand why people think and behave as they do is to realize that to anyone else, you are not the most important. They are.

Even knowing I wasn't alone, and that this predicament was permanent, I still found myself waffling through approach-avoidance tendencies. The frightening images of such a radical operation yanked my emotions to and fro. You could say I became a human yo-yo. One day I'd be resigned to the idea of surgery. The next morning I'd be limping as fast as an arthritic hip could carry me away from choosing this drastic operation. Then, one afternoon while trailing behind a

grocery shopping cart (a.k.a. Mike's rolling walker), another friend named Fran
Alexander eased up behind and startled
me by yelling out for everyone in the store
to hear: "Hello there, crip."

Fran had undergone traditional hip
replacement two years earlier. That day
she was literally waltzing smooth and
graceful circles around me flashing an
ear-to-ear grin. "When are you going to
face the music and get it done?" She was
reveling in her superior position. "You
know that until you suck it up and do it
like I had to, you are only going to get
worse. Things won't improve until you get
that bad hip replaced and begin to heal.
Just look at me now." She continued her
graceful little dance with that aggravat-
ing wide smile.

Actually, I had to chuckle at her good-natured teasing. Yet inside, I knew her candid assessment was right on target. Intellectual honesty told me my condition was doomed to only worsen with time. There was quite literally no hope for improvement until I faced reality. Finally, I summoned the moxie to make an appointment with Dr. Duke Harris, one of this booming region's most experienced orthopedic surgeons.

A friendly and engaging man, he had performed thousands of successful hip replacements over the years using the traditional method. I carried my initial X-ray from the general practitioner's office to our appointment. His office staff made a second film for comparison. Naturally, I had quietly hoped that a miracle healing had transpired since the initial diagnosis.

In my mind's eye, I visualized him examining his latest X-Ray, dropping his jaw in amazement, exclaiming: "Oh my God, Mike, it's a miracle. Why, I've never seen anything like this in 30 years of medicine. Your hip joint has somehow regrown enough cartilage and fluid to become normal once more. Why, it may even be better than normal. Have you been bathing at Lourdes?"

Yeah, dream on Mike, you increasingly hipless wonder. Instead, the physician kindly backhanded my cheek with the damned icy glove of reality. The truth was that the arthritis had become even more advanced inside my joint, leaving only the barest trace of any remaining cartilage. "I'd say you have another six months to a year before you can't use that leg much at all," he said. "You could have the replacement surgery right now. But it's really up to you to decide. In the end, it really all boils down to just how much pain you're willing to endure and for how long."

Then he demonstrated the metallic and plastic implants he'd been installing for years. He explained how in surgery he would carve a 10 to 12-inch incision down the length of my right hip, slicing through the muscles to fully access the diseased joint. Two hours later, he'd be stitching me up, applying pressure stockings to discourage possible blood clots and sending me off to post-operative care and months of recovery.

He explained that I could expect to spend at least four days in the hospital following surgery, perhaps followed by a few more evenings in a rehabilitation facility. "You'll be on a walker or crutches for the first six weeks after surgery without bearing weight at all on your operated hip," he said. "Then I'll let you use a cane until you are walking steadily. There likely won't be any driving a vehicle for about seven or eight weeks." My heart sank into my left heel.

I walked outside into the afternoon sun a few minutes later with that familiar edginess churning in my gut. The surgery he'd described sounded about as appealing as choking down a pound of cold, raw liver. I felt twinges of self pity and panic. There was that anger welling once again. "Why me? Where did this crap come from in the first place?" I mumbled aloud, climbing behind the steering wheel. "I was doing fine for such a long time and then, wham, I'm faced from out of nowhere with making this kind of decision. I'm too busy and I've got too many demands on me to deal with this." Then I remembered the words of my late father when he told me, "There's nothing about our lives, son, that carries a fairness clause."

Short of living with this painful affliction, what choice was there? Absolutely none. It also was anything but reassuring to bump into an emergency room physician at the Fayetteville Athletic Club later that day. He listened patiently to my tale of woe and expressed sympathy with my lack of choices. "Well, I know that hip replacement surgery can be a real hog killing," he said shaking his head. The good doctor could have gone the rest of his life - and mine for that matter - without implanting that barnyard-awful image. Despite the vision of some bloody swine spread-eagled and squealing across an operating table, I reluctantly wound up scheduling my very own "hog-killing" with Dr. Harris for six weeks from that day.

The Bargaining

That evening I prayed intently for divine intervention as I had done almost every night since learning of my predicament. "Please let me awaken and discover all this has been nothing but a bad dream," the pleas tumbled out freely. "Let me awake and be healed in the morning. I know such things have happened to others when they have sought your help. Why, I know you've even cured blind people." Then, as happens whenever we open our eyes and truly listen to the gentle breezes of consciousness continuously swirling around and through us, the whispers of higher awareness flowed in to intervene in mine.

A few days after I'd surrendered to the traditional replacement surgery, Hector Cueva, a colleague and friend, mentioned he'd seen a TV program the night before about a revolutionary new surgical technique for replacing hips. "I can't remember what the procedure is called or much about it except they said the incisions are a lot smaller and recovery is lots easier and faster," he said. "I immediately thought of you." As with others, Hector had watched my golf game rapidly degenerate along with my hip into a stumbling shadow of what it had been just a year earlier.

I returned to the keyboard and the Internet where I typed in "hip replacement surgery." In moments, a lengthy list appeared on the monitor, which included a reference to the Zimmer method and its revolutionary form of "minimally invasive arthroplasty." My heart leapt as I read how a limited number of surgeons nationwide in the past year had started using two different muscle and tendon-sparing techniques for replacing hips.

They could accomplish a replacement using either dual, two-inch surgical cuts, or a single 3-to-4 inch incision. They used various hip prostheses, identical to traditional replacements, only they inserted the devices via these mini-incisions with the help of specialized instruments and skills developed by the Zimmer Corporation of Indiana.

Actually, it turns out the methods were developed within the past decade by a surgeon in Chicago who began by performing the muscle-sparing surgery on cadavers.

The approach seemed so much more civilized and preferable to the traditional replacement. In fact, I read how patients of the Zimmer approach often were back on their feet and actually bearing weight on their operated hips within days of surgery. Some reported being mobile without support in less than two weeks. I devoured the material. Then I began trying to locate a surgeon nearby who might be skilled in this unique procedure.

Finally I gave up my Internet search and simply telephoned the Zimmer corporation in search of a physicians list and pamphlet. At that time, I didn't realize fewer than 300 surgeons worldwide were trained in their new method. A week later the promised Zimmer brochure arrived. Even more significant, a second letter sent by the office of Dr. William F. Hefley Jr. located three hours south in Little Rock, sat beside it in the mailbox.

It turned out that Dr. Hefley at that time was one of only two surgeons in three surrounding states who was qualified to use Zimmer's sophisticated techniques and equipment. And in what I saw as yet another subtle whisper from somewhere around me, he just happened to be listed

as an approved provider on our company's
health insurance plan.

I made an appointment for the following week. But then those nagging
doubts began to creep in. I had read
about how the dual, two-inch method,
which separated muscles and tendons
rather than slicing through them, likely
could not be performed on larger people
(like me). I started to rationalize that I
was wasting my time by even feeling the
slightest twinges of hope.

While my surgery at that time still
had been scheduled for six weeks later
with Dr. Harris, I noticed how Dr. Hefley's
name kept strangely cropping up amongst
those I knew, as well as with complete
strangers in unexpected moments. I'd

be talking in a group somewhere and the next thing I'd know, someone would be telling of a friend who'd had "the new hip replacement surgery done in Little Rock." I came to perceive all these messages as subtle urgings toward placing me where I was supposed to be. So I made an appointment with Dr. Hefley and drove to Little Rock with my sweetheart companion and best friend Judith Evans.

Inside his comfortable and jam-packed Little Rock office, Dr. Hefley's staff made yet a third X-Ray of my hip. Then he and his physician's assistant, Ken Weaver, both examined my expanding portfolio of charts and films to reach the same conclusion. Sure enough, my right hip still needed replacing.

As Dr. Hefley methodically conducted his physical examination to determine if I was a candidate for his technique, a form of peace settled around me like a velvet cape laid across my shoulders. I truly felt this place and this person, finally, was where I was led to be.

Dr. Hefley and his physician's assistant, seemed confident I would do well through the surgery, although he methodically described every possible risk. Hearing about the risks, a necessity for any surgeon to protect them from the lawyer's scalpel, is never all that reassuring. It turns out, I had less than a one in 100 chance of developing most of the potential complications he reviewed with me.

I asked if he could perform the dual-incision method, which I knew could completely spare my hip muscles, ligaments and tendons from being severed. He and Weaver agreed that method might be possible, especially if I could shed 20 pounds between then and surgery day. I set that date for two months later on Nov. 11. But he wanted me to know that even at my new and improved reduced weight, I'd still be the largest of his patients ever to undergo the dual-incision method. "We will see how it goes between now and then," he said, smiling. That was good enough for me.

I realized that at 264 pounds and six-feet tall, I had some heavy lifting ahead of me for that method to become a possibility. So, I went back home, canceled my

surgery with Dr. Harris and began exercising in the athletic club pool five times a
week. I found that even with a bad hip, I
could rapidly walk up to a mile each day in
the waist-deep water, while using webbed
pool gloves to strengthen my upper body.
This would become my daily routine over
the next eight weeks as the pounds thankfully began melting away and strength began to increase.

The Despair

While I was feeling more optimistic and healthier than I had in months, I began experiencing all forms of strange excuses rooted in fear. Despair and some anger began creeping into my thoughts, especially late at night. They went something like: "What if I have complications afterwards? It is a long drive to Little Rock when they could perform one of those traditional "hog killings" right here. I wondered what kind of surgeon this Dr. Hefley really was?

During the predawn hours as the days ticked away, I'd often awaken in a fretty sweat over the pending surgery. My mind would race to that one in a hundred possibility of complications from a possible blood clot to an infection, or even an accidental hip dislocation. I found myself rationalizing that *someone* had to be that unfortunate 100th patient. And with Mikey's Law in effect all these years, it would most likely be me.

The fear sometimes also would send me into a tailspin of situational depression and despair as I pondered the uncertainty of what awaited. In those darkest nights I came to understand how fear is truly humankind's greatest debilitator. We so easily become obsessed in its grasp for reasons not rooted in logic or common sense.

And its strangling fingers often clamp tightly around the neck of our hope and vitality where they squeeze until every drop of joy and hope is wrung completely away. But I also realized as time passed that perhaps, just maybe mind you, there was reason to banish that fear and become optimistic. I wanted to believe how dramatically the quality of my daily life would improve once this surgery was behind me.

The Acceptance

After boiling it continuously inside my head and sacrificing hours of precious sleep, the conclusion was always the same: This must be done if I'm ever to improve. And when I finally reached that point after weeks of prolonged back and forth bargaining, the tensions did ease. I even began to view my impending surgery as another of life's adventures.

I saw that I could choose to live the rest of my life as the partial cripple I'd become, or restore the fullest possible quality of life I had enjoyed for the first 56 years. And the answer was always a no-brainer. It was within the black and white boundaries of that conclusion that I slowly resigned myself to having total hip replacement surgery and the promise it held for my remaining years.

The periods of backsliding into fear and anger steadily dissolved, re-emerging only briefly to tease me with denial. For instance, I remember laying beside Judith one evening about two weeks before my surgery. I was in that yo-yoing denial mode for the 50th time, prompting me to blurt out in the darkness: "Maybe I'll just cancel this surgery. I mean I really don't have to go through this as long as I can still walk."

I felt her gazing toward me before softly responding: "But Michael, that's the point. You can't walk." I silently pondered the honesty of her words until I accepted truth once again and sleep overcame me.

Having published several earlier newspaper columns about my struggle to overcome osteoarthritis through exercise and pills, I would come to write three in particular that described my pre-surgery anxieties, the surgery, itself, and the aftereffects two weeks later.

I had hoped many others who would one-day face this same decision might find

comfort in my deeply personal experiences. The initial column told of being es-
corted into surgery at the Baptist Health
Medical Center in Little Rock after resist-
ing that moment for over a year. I wrote
about how my most determined efforts to
defeat the disease had led to this harsh
reality. And I quoted a lifelong friend as
comparing my damaged hip to a vehicle's
"worn out ball joint."

Readers of my column learned
how, for 56 years I somehow had avoided
spending a single night in a hospital bed.
And they read how I had discovered comfort in simply realizing I wasn't alone in
my affliction. Scores of thousands in our
50's today can expect to have joints replaced as the scourge of osteoarthritis
cripples us over the coming years. In fact,

my understanding is at least 300,000 hip replacement surgeries already are being performed across America each year.

"Some of you know from previous columns that I have fought the relentless disease that took root and began growing several years ago," I wrote in the initial essay. "My primary weapons were prescription pain pills, diet and supervised exercise at the Fayetteville Athletic Club. But the beast gnawing away down there laughed out loud at everything I fired as it continued gorging on the natural cushions inside my joint. But guess who's getting the last laugh?"

I then described how my limp had worsened into almost a shuffle and how dragging my leg for days on end had kept me continually worn out. I grew weary of feeling as if I was still 30 in many ways while hobbling as though I were 80.

My natural hip joint will be replaced with a high-tech cobalt /chrome and ir-radiated polyethylene version, I also told readers. The pre-surgery tests were com-pleted at Baptist Health Medical Center where each hospital nurse and technician took turns poking, attaching, X-raying and even turning the tables to interview me, the journalist. Finally, I was pronounced fit to assume center gurney beneath the lights with Dr. William Hefley and crew.

The difference between the tradi-tional hip replacement and the Zimmer approach was the comparison between up to a 13-inch vertical cut through my hip muscle with either a single three-inch slice or dual two-inch incisions in which the muscles, tendons and ligaments are spared the knife.

Both Zimmer minimal incision techniques also greatly reduce most patients' rehabilitation period as well as the scar size. A traditional hip replacement without complications can mean about four days in the hospital, followed by perhaps a few more in a rehabilitation facility.

I'd also been told to expect six weeks on crutches without placing the slightest weight on the affected hip. I learned that, barring complications, many Zimmer-method patients are on their feet within hours of surgery and often discharged from the hospital within 24 hours.

There also is not a formal rehabilitation, that column further explained, except for a self-directed exercise program with the Zimmer method. Patients are encouraged to put as much weight as they are comfortable with on their new hip as soon as possible. In fact Dr. Hefley told me this hip replacement method, now less than two years old, is evolving toward becoming same-day outpatient surgery. Driving to Little Rock to have this technique seemed far preferable.

Dr. Hefley, a Vanderbilt Medical School graduate and father of four, initially told me that performing the dual two-inch method on a person my size would be a challenge. The procedure seemed to work best on thinner people with small to mid-sized bones. If he agreed to utilize this procedure with my hip, I'd become his largest dual-incision patient.

Yet he had agreed at our first session seven weeks earlier that if I could shed 20 pounds before surgery, he might attempt it, rather than the single, mini-incision, which usually requires a slightly longer recovery period. "I had managed to drop 16 pounds by surgery day.," I explained in that particular column. "I'll know when I awaken later this morning, which technique he selected."

Actually, because I had written the surgery column beforehand out of necessity, he would inform me of his final decision as I was about to head for the operating room. "It was reassuring to hear him tell me on the day before surgery that his primary concern was to provide me with the best hip possible that would serve me well for at least 20 years," I wrote in the column.

I should insert here that several hundred surgeons worldwide are now performing the Zimmer-technique. I happened to discover Dr. Hefley in Little Rock and am writing here of my personal experiences with him. But the growing number of surgeons that Dr. Hefley and other pioneers of the method are educating, can be equally competent and effective in my opinion.

I'm simply saying that with a computer and a phone book, anyone can likely find a Zimmer minimally-invasive surgeon within driving distance who can evaluate their unique needs and hopefully offer the same advantages I discovered.

I recall asking one of Dr. Hefley's experienced nurses during an early office visit if it was normal for prospective re-placees to be feeling nervous and even re-morseful at the thought of giving up their natural hip joint. After all, it was the hip that had carried them through thousands of miles of walking, running, jumping and such. She smiled and explained that such concerns are most natural for patients, especially among younger ones.

Most older patients have been living in agonizing pain for so long, that they just want relief, she said. Afterwards, she added, patients say the artificial replacement feels as natural as their other good hip. "It will be nice to realize what it once felt like not to have this constant pain," I wrote in a column.

A lifelong friend, Don Walker, later would remind me how his artificially implanted teeth worked great. Judith and my daughter, Anna, said they've functioned very well for years without their appendixes. Four others with hips replaced by Dr. Hefley, sang an identical chorus. This surgery supposedly had been the best thing that had happened to them since their hips began failing. And each person said their recoveries all had gone even better than they'd hoped or expected.

The number of hip replacement surgeries, as well as other joints like knees, is skyrocketing each year. Dr. Hefley, who utilizes surgical suites at both the Baptist Health Medical Center and St. Vincent's Medical Center in Little Rock medical centers, recently performed 17 hip replacements in one week. He, alone, is now doing about 400 hip replacements a year. And he explained that, while he still performs more of the single mini-incision operations, the number of two-incision replacements is steadily increasing.

"Hopefully, today's words as well as those in future columns that describe this method of hip replacement surgery, might serve to comfort many others who one day will join the club. I'll be back soon on crutches to tell you what the surgery experience itself was like," I wrote in the column leading up to my operation.

Included on my list of pre-opera-
tion "to-do" instructions was a daily iron
tablet beginning three weeks before
surgery. It's truly remarkable how much
iron tastes on the human tongue like the
metal it is, even when I hurried it's journey to the stomach with a single gulp. I
always tried swallowing mine with some
food to prevent the possibility of an upset
stomach.

I also found myself in the month
before surgery, lying face-up on a local
Red Cross gurney pumping a rubber ball
and trying not to watch as the technician
painlessly inserted the needle. Dr. Hefley
needed two units of my own blood to use
as needed after surgery. I had a month

to schedule and keep two presurgery appointments, which I did.

Actually, giving blood wasn't that bad. Other than the pages of paperwork to complete before the needle was inserted, I found the process to be relatively painless. The cookies and juice afterwards actually made me feel like I was being rewarded like a dutiful second grader for having done something good.

The Red Cross also took care to ensure my blood was correctly identified before shipping it to Little Rock to await my arrival. I even signed the backside of the bag and agreed to have nurses on surgery day double check the units for accuracy. Those kind of precautions only made me feel better.

On the weekend before the big day, Judith and I held a "Kiss Mike's Hip Good-bye" party on the backyard patio. All our friends showed up for the festivities and to offer moral support. Today, I believe I recall one or two actually kissing that bad hip, or at least the material of my slacks that covered it that evening.

That was one evening I also kissed my Type II diabetes goodbye for a few hours and struck up a much closer relationship with old friend, Jim Beam. I figured if I'd ever toasted to anything, it might as well have been to the many years of good service the original right hip had provided me.

I recall everyone assuring me that all would go well with the operation. In fact most said they had not "even one negative concern" about what I was about to do. As I've aged, I have tended to put more stock in the intuitions we all feel about ourselves and those we care about. So their words of encouragement were comforting.

A few days following the operation, in a column entitled: "One Hip Day in the OR," I sat at the keyboard to describe the details of this surgical experience that I'd dreaded for so long.

Inside the OR

"It was Tuesday, November 11 at 5:30 a.m. The sun was still an hour from rising on this Veteran's Day as the automatic doors at Baptist Health Medical Center in Little Rock whisked open," I wrote in that piece. " I limped inside with a bad case of butterflies and cotton mouth. Within three hours, my arthritic right hip joint would be replaced with cobalt chrome and irradiated polyethylene. I drew long, deep breaths hoping no one would notice my swelling anxiety.

Yet the troubling uncertainties of a surgical virgin continued churning deep in my gut as a smiling lady at the front desk politely took my name. She directed me toward a lobby seat with five others also awaiting the scalpel that morning. Without knowing their names, I felt an instant bond with these somber-faced men and women.

Within a few minutes, a man whose shirt badge read "Willie" arrived. He began calling our names and checking his cards. Then, in a move that reminded me of boot camp, he instructed us to follow him in a group. We were heading back to the pre-surgery ward where we would be prepared for our operations. We followed quietly behind Willie, each of us absorbed in our own thoughts. We'd been warned of the risks and potential complications of our various surgeries. We had signed our approvals. Now reality hour was rapidly approaching.

At one hallway crossroads, Willie unexpectedly directed our accompanying support groups of family and friends into the crowded surgical waiting room where some were sleeping on couches. I hugged Judith, handed her my watch and ring, then watched her head toward the open door. The pale and slender young man beside me told me he was about to have a cancerous kidney removed. His fight sparked resolve inside me at the right moment. Wishing each other well, we stepped into the vast prep room.

Inside that chilly area, Willie handed us warmed white blankets and pointed us toward hospital beds inside glass-fronted, two-bed rooms that lined the ward. "Lay on your back and cover up with this blanket," Willie said. I followed his instructions, depositing my clothes into a plastic bag, donning the goofy open-backed hospital gown and feeling the blanket's comfortable warmth as I lay quietly staring at the stark ceiling for the next 15 minutes.

Outside the room, I could hear the bustle of nurses and technicians chatting and laughing as they carried out another workday. For them, this was just one more day on the clock with patients they did not know and likely would never see again. For us, however, these were anxious, uncertain minutes over what the coming hours and years would bring. A person can do a lot of soul searching while lying alone in that anxious hour before major surgery.

Those few reflective moments quickly faded into a whirlwind of nurses and technicians. They were arriving to draw blood, shave my lower right side and connect the IV line into the top of my right hand. A friendly nursing student walked in and said she'd be "shadowing my case" from beginning to end for a class paper. My amiable anesthesiologist also named Mike, whom I was meeting for the first time, strolled in with a grin. His casual sense of humor actually put me at ease for the first time that morning.

The pain-numbing epidural he was about to insert into the middle of my spinal column as I sat hunched over on the skinny bed would be the most unpleasant experience of my stay. It wasn't that the procedure was that painful. Rather, it was wondering just what the heck he was doing back there - and knowing this device would remain inserted throughout my hospital stay.

If you've ever been stung by a wasp or flipped with a rubber band you've felt what it's like to have an epidural inserted. Bam, ouch and it's gone. The initial discomfort quickly became a memory. I laid back, drew a few more deep breaths, and began to notice the effects of the numbing medication that was dripping slowly into my body from two bags. Others who had been through this surgery had correctly predicted how I would quickly come to appreciate both the calming and numbing effects of an epidural. Now I finally understood why they use these things in childbirth.

In a matter of minutes, I didn't even care if they removed my thinking head, much less my femoral head. Momentarily, Dr. Hefley's new surgical assistant. David Gibson, was standing over me grinning and reassuring that everything would go well. Ken Weaver had been called up as a medic with his Guard unit for duty in Iraq.

Then Dr. Hefley appeared, also wearing a broad smile. Does everyone here just smile a lot? I recall wondering. When I'd left Dr. Hefley the previous afternoon, he was still pondering whether he could successfully pull off the dual, two-inch incision technique on someone six-feet-tall and weighing 246 pounds.

The decision was between that method or the three-inch single mini-incision he generally used for larger people. The difference in these two Zimmer techniques can amount to only an extra week or so of recovery, because the single incision method usually requires a relatively small cut through a portion the hip muscle.

Hovering over me, Dr. Hefley said that after thoughtful consideration and consultation, he was going with the two-incisions. Now I was grinning from ear to ear, feeling especially thankful that I'd worked so hard to drop those extra pounds.

A nurse then placed the silver ex-panding surgical beret over my head and we began rolling my conglomeration of poles, tubes and bags down the hallway and toward kickoff. After years of limp-ing and shuffling, all those pills, months of workouts in a swimming pool, and so many midnight anxieties over this mo-ment, it finally was game time.

Laying there, I also recalled the words of my favorite uncle named Ken Mas-terson who, at 74, had undergone several major surgeries of his own over the years:

"Mike," he'd told me, "believe me, all those worries you feel before anything even happens will be the worst part of the experience."

Sure enough, there wasn't a trace of anxiety by the time I rolled into that expansive and frigid surgical suite. I noticed a half dozen people in bluish gowns mingling and arranging glistening whatevers. There were trays of what appeared to be mechanic's parts near the operating table. Dr. Hefley and the Zimmer representative were waiting to begin the show. As with other prosthetic manufacturers, Zimmer has a representative in surgery to assist in constructing a customized hip for each patient.

I later learned that a skilled manufacturer's representative is a vital partner to have in surgery, considering there are thousands of potential choices of parts from which a physician can choose in reconstructing a human hip joint. It seems the sizes of our hip balls and sockets can vary widely, based on a person's body and bone sizes.

They also often insert a couple of screws into the hard plastic cup to make certain it holds firmly in place inside the bone, exactly as they were about to do with me. A few men on the surgical team helped slide me sideways from the gurney onto the operating table.

Seemingly from out of the woodwork, two younger men, both also named

Mike, were standing above me. One placed a clear plastic mask over my nose saying, "We're going to give you a little oxygen. Now were giving you a little gas, so just breathe deeply and relax," added the other Mike. I remember wondering how confusing it could be to have a dozen or so of us Mike's in the operating room. As I quickly drifted off, I wondered how that young fellow with kidney cancer was doing with his surgery, and how precious Judith was faring out in that crowded waiting room.

In but an 'Instant'

"In what literally seemed like the next instant, I was hearing beeps and a gentle voice asking: 'Mr. Masterson, can you hear me? Are you awake? Your hip replacement surgery is over and you did just fine,'" I wrote in the column. I opened my eyes to a nurse who was checking vital signs in the post-operative recovery room. There were others in similar beds around the spacious room. My surgery that had lasted two hours was seemingly over in only a blink of my life.

Both legs were tightly strapped to a pillow wedged between them. That was to keep my fresh hip from moving. I needed no IV narcotic to control pain. Dr. Hefley opts for the epidural and pain pills as needed rather than knocking his patients cold with hard narcotics. This method of pain control also enables his post-operative patients to become active much more quickly than if they remain dazed by harder drugs.

Ninety minutes later I was arriving in room 310. There, I quickly met a seemingly endless flow of nurses and hospital staff. Each of them would play a role in helping make my life more comfortable over the next 23 hours. During the previous year, Baptist Health alone had seen and cared for 500 knee and 325 total hip replacement patients. And one national publication recently had named it the hospital of choice in Little Rock for ortho-pedic surgeries and treatment. I felt like I was in the right place.

Dr. Hefley stopped by my room to say the replacement he'd just completed on me had exceeded even his most hope-ful expectations. This success also had encouraged him to attempt the two-in-cision method on other larger patients, which helped me understand how it had served a purpose much larger than my own needs.

Immediately after surgery, Dr. Hef-ley had hurried the X-Ray of my new hip into the waiting room where he proudly held it to the light to show Judith. That X-Ray provides the cover for this book. The dark metallic rod and ball and the new hard-plastic cup stood in dark contrast to the lighter natural bone encasing it. Compared with X-rays taken previously of my diseased hip, this newer model looked tight and well-fitted, although unnaturally odd resting with two prominent screws amidst the other more-faded images.

In the following hours in Room 310, I discovered that post-surgical patients shouldn't plan on sleeping much during their first night in the hospital. The nurses have their hourly responsibilities - all those temperatures and blood pressures and IV connections to check and thick charts to maintain. Before midnight they'd paid at least a dozen visits, which roused me each time. But I did manage to doze several hours between midnight and 7 a.m. when the nursing shift changed.

In my ignorance, I was unprepared to urinate into a hand-held plastic urinal while lying flat on my back and numbed from the belly button down. But urinate you must unless, of course, you prefer having a plastic catheter rudely installed into the place where that routinely occurs. I opted with the assistance of two nurses aides to get myself vertical beside the bed and partially stand on my new hip eight hours after surgery. The last thing I wanted was to enjoy the astonishing pleasures of a catheter installation.

The next morning, the nursing staff aroused me to remove the IV and the drainage tube from my front incision. I didn't feel either one. They also changed my bandages once again and said everything looked fine. Hearing those words brought another sigh of relief. I was now past the surgery phase and into the "fear of possible complications" period.

The two strapping guys who'd saved me from the catheter during the previous afternoon arrived to stand me upright once again and hand me that walker. I used it to ease down the hallway to the Occupational Therapy ward. There, the staff spent over an hour helpfully teaching me the medically correct way to sit, shower, climb stairs, conduct the necessary business of toiletry and use crutches and the walker. It all seemed like common sense. Yet they dutifully handed over diagrams and directions for those who preferred to study the details in depth.

Gone in 23 hours

The bottom line of all my months of worry and fear? Less than 24 hours after entering the hospital room, two nurses named Otto and Kim were rolling me out to the curb in a wheelchair for the three-hour ride back to Fayetteville. The only difficult period in that journey came when nature called and we stopped along a dirt road so I could stand and deliver. I probably could have even avoided that rather unpleasant inconvenience if

I'd simply remembered to use that plastic urinal packed inside my suitcase.

It's also germane to report that I only took one prescription pain pill as a precaution for that journey. And I really didn't feel like I even needed that medication.

Three days after surgery, I was bearing nearly full weight on my operated hip using a walker and was even able to stand balanced and freely on both legs for more than a minute without much discomfort or support. The gnawing pain that had resided for so long inside my groin and hip joint had instantly vanished immediately after surgery. Others who had been through the operation had told me the discomfort would be gone when I awoke.

Dr. Hefley told me I would be walking on a cane in less than 10 days and back to taking a full shoulder turn on the golf course in fewer than 12 weeks. My friends who may be about to join the hip replacee's club may wonder if I'd choose this surgical method again after my experiences?

Without a millimeter of hesitation - or fear. So my advice based on my experience is to grit your teeth and get your precious mobility back. And remember the late John Denver when he advised us how those things we fear at the most mean nothing. And just look, everything that worried him in his relatively brief life really amounted to nothing in the end, didn't it?

My 'After Experience'

Below, I've provided some additional observations about my post-surgical experiences offered solely from one patient's point of view. Hopefully, my experiences can help you make solid choices for your own life.

Removing the staples on the eighth day was nothing at all - no pain - barely a tweak. I shouldn't have wasted a second concerning myself with that process. I didn't feel all that good about taking the daily blood thinner medication prescribed to help prevent a blood clot. Taking rat poison just seemed so unnatural.

But I swallowed the stuff anyway and paid regular weekly visits to the general practitioner to ensure my bloodstream was reflecting properly diluted levels. Those visits lasted five weeks. I was told that I couldn't consume cabbage or take vitamins during that period because nutrients high in Vitamin K can negate the effects of the blood thinner.

At bedtime, I had to sleep either on my back, or on my the un-operated side. It didn't feel natural and interfered with my rest for a while. I also kept a pillow tucked well into my groin and another for my feet to keep my legs separated while laying on my side. This lasted about a month. It is difficult to get comfortable sleeping only on your back or on the same side. But I became more accustomed to the drill after about a week. The first few nights, I spent parts of each night sleeping in my new lift-recliner, which may have been the most comfortable place of all. You'll need one.

I also took naps to try and stay caught up on my rest, since I'm one who needs about eight hours of sleep a night to feel even remotely rested. Sleeping, or rather the lack of it, was my greatest adjustment in the weeks immediately following the operation.

I got up to go to the bathroom and move around at least 40 or 50 steps every waking hour or so during that first week. And I made it a point to keep moving my feet and flexing my thigh muscles whenever I sat in a chair. I planned on spending the first four days at home walking as it felt right and using a walker for support, but also taking it easy, if that makes much sense. I didn't want to set myself back a week or so by overdoing in that first week.

I'd found and purchased an aluminum walker for $7 at the same junk and bait shop where I also bought worms for my backyard pond fish. They also had a good pair of metal crutches for $7, so I'd added them to the arsenal.

My operated leg felt as weak as overcooked spaghetti for the first couple of days. But I found those muscles were re-gaining strength at the rate of about five percent a day over the first week. That daily gain slowed to two or three percent in subsequent weeks. But it was always steadily improving until by the end of the third week, I was walking without a cane or a walker. Yet I frequently used the cane so as not to overstrain.

By the beginning of the third week, I'd become strong enough in my operated leg to easily drive a car, as long as I took my time entering and exiting. I sometimes forgot to keep my leg in the proper position, which triggered a sharp reminder. That, of course, was always followed by the certainty that I probably had managed to dislocate my new hip.

Thankfully, that proved to be a mis-assumption. It seems I'd only aggravated those tender and healing muscles and tendons with those sudden moves and thrusts.

In the weeks immediately follow-ing surgery, I focused whenever reclined or seated on moving my feet continuously back and forth and up and down at the ankles to keep blood circulating properly. My greatest fear was the formation of a blood clot and this was a way, other than standing and moving regularly, to help prevent one.

The muscles in my operated-side buttocks and outer thigh remained some-what tender for several weeks, which I'd expected. They seemed tight and, well, balled up. Placing heat pads across them helped loosen the discomfort. While my knee was fine, other patients told me their operated-side knee muscles had remained unusually tight and somewhat sore for several months after surgery. The remedy they'd discovered was to actually use-and thereby stretch out-those taut muscles.

My front 2.5-inch incision wasn't healed as much as I hoped to see until the end of the third week. I was pleased to see the hot-pink-colored drain incision had completed its purpose and scabbed over well. By the fourth week, the pinkness was diminishing and it was obvious I was healing very well in that area.

The smaller rear incision had sealed over quickly without much discoloration. That front cut just took longer because that is where the surgeon had inserted the deep surgical drain tube. I made sure to keep the wound clean and dry by using a blow dryer set on low heat. The tissues around the front incision and down into my thigh remained somewhat numb during these initial weeks, which in looking back I can see was just part of the healing process.

I began liberally applying hydrogen peroxide to that front wound during the second week. But that seemed to only keep it more inflamed looking, a condition that began to disappear as soon as I quit using the stuff and simply bathed the cut daily with antibacterial soap and water.

A hand-held shower is a must. I'd keep the operated side of my body outside the shower curtain while rinsing down the other side. Then I'd cut the water off, lather up and shampoo on the good side before rinsing. I spent the first 10 days using a wash cloth to cleanse the operated half of my body. That seemed to work fine.

After a few weeks , I stood inside the free-standing stall to take a normal shower, always using a blow dryer to air dry the incisions. That technique seemed to work well, except for the morning when my operated leg slid suddenly sideways on a slick, wet floor, causing a sharp hip-area pain and another of those "oh-no" moments.

During another second - week adventure, I plopped into a hard-backed chair with such force that it splintered and collapsed, spilling me onto the tile kitchen floor. Thankfully, my operated side leg had been extended when the fall came, rather than bent beneath me.

The most challenging part of that sudden drop onto the tile was trying to regain my feet without bending the operated-side knee. What a sight those three minutes must have been. With Judith's help, I finally regained my feet and spent the remainder of the day in close proximity to the security of that $7 bait-shop walker.

Frankly, I was anxious to get back to regularly exercising in a swimming pool, which required that both surgical wounds be fully sealed over. Then I thought about all those traditional hip surgery replacees who had to remain on crutches for at least six full weeks. And I quickly felt much better.

I've come to believe that working out in a pool, even if it is just rapid walking back and forth, complimented with webbed exercise gloves for upper body workout, is the best for me. It takes all weight off my hip while working and strengthening the related muscles, tendons and ligaments. I was back to my water routine by the fourth week.

There were up and down days mentally and emotionally immediately following surgery. I knew going into the experience that the six weeks after my operation would be the most demanding in every respect. And they were. But it wasn't all bad by any stretch of my expectations. I just had some, well, I suppose I'd call them the *grayer days* when I just wanted it all to just hurry up and get better. After three full weeks, I felt like I was definitely on the mend and bound for normal walking over the remainder of my life.

The fact that my hip was "artificial" by then seemed irrelevant. I'd become results-oriented. The day-by-day improvement had left me feeling so much better that the "how" of all this didn't matter nearly as much as in those anxious, uncertain days before surgery.

And, while I'm sharing so much personal information, why not step to the plate right here and address the issue of sexual relations. One problem with arthritis in either hip is that the grinding internal pain reeks havoc with more than one's mobility. Let's say it affects your mobility in a number of endeavors. But that disease pain vanished with the surgery.

By the fifth week, there were many evenings when we both would conclude shared affections with mutual whispers: "Thank you, Dr. Hefley." In more direct terms, yes my friends in the aftermath of hip replacement, there is pain-free, highly-mobile sex. In fact there were times when I swore I was 15 again.

Following the columns in the *Arkansas Democrat-Gazette*, my telephone began ringing regularly with inquiries from others who were suffering with osteoarthritis. I understood their fears and feelings because I once had been exactly where they were at that moment. They asked many of the same questions I'd had beforehand and have answered in this little book. One caller was particularly interested in restoring two aspects of life: sex with his wife and snow skiing.

"You think I'll be able to do both of those things again if I have this done?" he asked. I responded that while I didn't ski, I felt if my experience was any indication, he could probably do that within reason. The surgeon certainly could answer that question. But as for the first part, I didn't need a doctor's advice or approval. "Man, that's some great news for me and for her," he said. "It's just been tough not being able to do what we both have wanted to do. This arthritis has really gotten me down." Yep, I could identify with his every word.

After 12 weeks, I was walking as normally as I ever had. And I was already preparing to hit the links with the arrival of Spring. The tenderness and those little lingering twinges of soreness and weakness in my thigh had vanished. The right hip actually felt solid. Even my virtually healed incisions were becoming little more than vague reminders that I'd ever had the operation. I'd describe it as blue skies returning. I felt myself anticipating the future rather than dwelling on what had been my incurable and hopeless predicament.

It was about this time that I chose to have my first professional massage on the tissues surrounding the affected hip. I felt both protective and apprehensive what that might be like to relax them fully. But after 45 minutes, I could tell it had done wonders for loosening up those muscles that had been tense and tight for so long in my hip and thigh. I was glad I'd invested the time and expense to have that done and I wished I'd had this massage after 10 weeks.

By four months out, all the tenderness had vanished and everything inside and around my right hip felt as solid as if I were 15 years old and running the 100-yard dash again at Harrison High School. Except Dr. Hefley tells me I can walk all I want, but not sprint or leap hurdles no matter how great I feel. It seems doing either would risk putting extreme force on the new hip and surrounding bone and tissues. And why in the world would I want to risk that?

During more philosophical moments, I've also lately started to compare this body of mine with a television or a radio created to temporarily receive signals of varying frequencies. Over time, parts of every set, exactly like our fragile bodies, invariably give out. Yet many also can now be replaced - for a while anyway until eventually their sole function ultimately fails for one cause or another. Yet the inevitable failure of our sets does not alter the constant signal they were created to receive.

Yes, we are comprised of parts that will wear out, whether they be hearts, lungs, knees, or hips. And the more weight we pack on over the years, the more pressures we place on them until they can no longer bear the load. Thankfully, the technology and human skills exist today (like the MIS hip replacement surgery) to replace so many of our exhausted organs and joints.

Some Final Thoughts

I am appreciative that my worn-out natural hip failed me at a time in history when replacing it could be such a relatively easy proposition. I'm told this surgery will soon even be utilizing the assistance of computers to match and fit every prostheses as perfectly as possible. In fact, computers already are being used with some such replacement surgeries nationwide.

Meanwhile, I've also adopted a new motto for overcoming life's crises. Hopefully, this message can serve every potential hip replacee and others who encounter the endless challenges of existence as well as it does me today: "Courage is not the absence of fear, but knowing that something is more important than fear."

If you're anything like I am, your heart, mind and gut know when the time has arrived to overcome your dread of this surgery, or any major surgery or obstacle, and move confidently toward restoring quality, satisfaction and vital purpose to your brief lifetime.

As I stated at the beginning, if this replacement were my decision to make again, I'd smile real wide, abandon all fear and dive into the experience headlong. The chill of uncertainty only lasts a moment. And, since this life we so desperately cling to is destined to be fragile and uncertain, regardless of whether or not we choose to worry about it, I'd also learn to trust in *uncertainty* itself.

We do come into this strange place alone and we depart by ourselves after making endless strings of choices during our stays. As with every challenge we inevitably face, my new hip has proven to be simply another choice, as well as a valuable learning experience in the overall process of living. More than anything, it is now a cause for hope as well as renewed quality of existence in what time remains. Here is to your quality of life - and to your greater understanding of what this surgery and the complex psychological and physical processes surrounding it were like - from one patient's perspective.

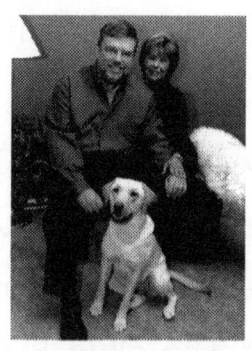

About the Author

Mike Masterson, 57, lives in Fay-etteville, Arkansas, where he writes up to four personal opinion columns each week as a full-time staff columnist for the statewide-circulated Arkansas Democrat-Gazette. His writing and reporting over the years has been nationally honored on more than two dozen occasions, including The George Polk Award, Four Robert F. Kennedy Awards, Two Heywood Broun Awards, Two Clarion Awards and twice he has been a finalist for the Pulitzer Prize. Mike also was an Alicia Patterson Fellow in 1976, and was the Kiplinger Professor and director of the Kiplinger Midcareer Program for Professional Journalists at The Ohio State University between 1989 and 1994. In addition to being editor of three Arkansas Daily newspapers over his 33-year career, he has been both a reporter and investigative editor for The Los Angeles Times, The Arizona Republic, The Chicago Sun-Times and the Asbury Park Press.